AF499088

# Table of Contents

## PREVIEW

Peripheral neuropathy refers to the conditions that result when nerves that carry messages to and from the brain and spinal cord from and to the rest of the body are damaged or diseased.

The peripheral nerves make up an intricate network that connects the brain and spinal cord to the muscles, skin, and internal organs. Peripheral nerves come out of the spinal cord and are arranged along lines in the body called dermatomes. Typically, damage to a nerve will affect one or more dermatomes, which can be tracked to specific areas of the body. Damage to these nerves interrupts communication between the brain and other parts of the body and can impair muscle movement, prevent normal sensation in the arms and legs, and cause pain.

# PERIPHERAL NEUROPATHY DIET RECIPES

## BREAKFAST

### 1. Black Bean Breakfast Burrito

Prep Time: 20 minutes

Cook Time: 45 minutes

Total Time: 1 hour 5 minutes

Servings: 2

## Ingredients

Pico de gallo:

- 1 plum tomato, seeded and diced
- 1 tablespoon finely chopped white or red onion
- 1 tablespoon minced jalapeño, deseeded
- 1 tablespoon fresh lime juice
- 1 tablespoon chopped cilantro
- Salt, to taste

Burrito:

- 4 large eggs
- Salt and pepper, to taste

- Pinch cayenne pepper (optional)
- 2 teaspoons canola or grape seed oil
- ⅓ cup grated Monterey Jack or Cheddar cheese
- 1 cup black beans, drained and rinsed
- 2 (9 inch) whole wheat tortillas
- ½ ripe avocado, peeled, pitted and diced

## Instructions

1. In a small bowl, mix together the diced tomato, onion, jalapeño, lime juice, cilantro, salt, and pepper. Set aside.
2. In a medium bowl, whisk the eggs with 1 teaspoon of water, cayenne pepper, if using, and salt and pepper.

3. In a medium non-stick skillet heat 1 teaspoon of oil over medium heat. Add the eggs and cook, stirring to scramble, just until set. Stir in in the cheese, and cook until all the cheese has melted. Remove from heat.

4. Wipe the same skillet clean. Heat the remaining 1 teaspoon of oil over medium-high heat, and add the drained black beans. Cook just until heated through, about 1 minute. Remove from heat.

5. Wipe the same skillet clean, and heat the tortillas, just until warmed.

6. Fill the tortillas vertically, across the center, with the pico de gallo, about an inch away from the edges. Then top with even amounts of beans, scrambled eggs, and diced avocado. Fold over the top and the bottom of the tortilla, then fold over the sides, overlapping them. Serve, folded side down.

## 2. Healthy Fruity Oatmeal

Prep Time: 15 minutes

Cook Time: 25 minutes

Total Time: 40 minutes

Servings: 10

Ingredients

- 1 ⅓ cups rolled oats (⅓ cup dry for 1 serving)
- 2 ⅔ cup water (⅔ cup water for ⅓ cup oatmeal)
- Generous pinch sea salt
- 1 tablespoon golden raisins
- 1 tablespoon dried cranberries
- ½ teaspoon cinnamon (optional)
- 2 apples
- 2 tablespoons sliced almonds, dry toasted
- 2 bananas, thinly sliced
- Milk of your choice, or yogurt to taste

Instructions

1. Mix the oats, water, salt, raisins, cranberries, and cinnamon in a pan. Bring to a boil, stir well and then lower the heat to a low simmer. Cook, covered, for

about 10 minutes, stirring the oatmeal from time to time so that it doesn"t stick.

2. While the oatmeal is cooking, grate the apple using the coarsest bore. When the oatmeal has cooked, stir in the grated apple until it is well mixed. Cover and turn the heat off. Leave the oatmeal for 5 minutes to steam. Serve sprinkled with almonds and sliced bananas, and with milk or yogurt on the side.

## 3. Kale & Mushroom Breakfast Sandwich

Prep Time: 15 minutes

Cook Time: 20 minutes

Total Time: 35 minutes

Servings: 2

Ingredients

- ¼ cup plain yogurt
- 2 tablespoons sriracha sauce
- 2 tablespoons olive oil
- 2 cup mushrooms, sliced
- 6 leaves kale, shredded
- salt and pepper to taste
- 2 eggs
- 4 slices whole wheat bread, toasted

Instructions

1. In a small bowl, mix together yogurt and sriracha.

2. Heat a sauté pan on medium heat. Add olive oil. Once hot, add the mushrooms and sauté for about 5 minutes, or until they start to turn golden brown. Add the kale along with about ¼ cup water. Cook until the

kale is wilted and the water has mostly evaporated. Season with salt and pepper.

3. Heat a greased non-stick pan on medium low heat. Crack and pour eggs into the pan. Cook until whites are set, flip and cook for 1 minute for a runny yolk, 3 minutes for a fully cooked yolk. Turn off the heat and let sit while assembling sandwich.

4. Place 2 slices of bread on 2 plates. Spread an even layer of the yogurt sauce over the toast. Top with a portion of kale, mushrooms and egg. Top with other slice of bread. Cut the sandwich down the middle and serve.

## 4. Quinoa With Roasted Ratatouille

Prep Time: 30 minutes

Cook Time: 35 minutes

Total Time: 1 hour 5 minutes

Servings: 6

Ingredients

- 2 tablespoons, plus 1 teaspoon, olive oil
- 2 cups Asian eggplant, 1 inch slices (if using the big Italian ones, cut into a 1 inch dice)
- 2 cups zucchini, cut into 1 inch chunks (if the zucchini are large, deseed them)
- 2 large red peppers, deseeded and cut into 1 inch pieces, about 2 cups
- 12 cloves of garlic in their skins (or to taste)
- 2 cups cherry tomatoes, washed and halved
- 2 cups quinoa, rinsed well in a fine sieve
- 4 cups water or stock
- 2 scallions, bottoms trimmed, greens kept and split lengthwise
- 3 tablespoons chopped Italian parsley, plus 1 sprig
- 3 shallots, thinly sliced

- ½ cup lightly packed torn basil leaves
- Sea salt, to taste

Instructions

1. Preheat the oven to 400 degrees.

2. Put 1 tablespoon of olive oil into a large bowl. Tip the eggplant, zucchini, red peppers, and garlic into the bowl and mix with your hands to coat them with oil. Spread them out in a single layer onto a couple of baking sheets. Sprinkle with sea salt. Tip the tomatoes into the bowl to coat with any remaining oil and add to the other vegetables, skin side down.

3. Roast the vegetables for 20 minutes on a high shelf. Turn with a spatula to mix and cook for another 10-15 minutes or until all the vegetables are soft, golden and caramelized around the edges. If the peppers cook faster than the rest, remove them from the tray and set aside.

4. While the vegetables are cooking, put the washed quinoa, parsley sprig, and scallions into a saucepan with a lid. Add the 4 cups of water and 1 tsp of olive oil

and bring to a boil. Cover, turn the heat to low and simmer for 15-20 minutes. Take off the heat and set aside, covered, until you are ready to use it.

5. While the quinoa is cooking, heat the remaining oil in a large pan over medium-low heat. When it starts to shimmer, add the shallots and sauté slowly until they turn golden and caramelized, about 8-10 minutes. Add the chopped parsley, cook for a minute and then, if they are ready, add the roasted vegetables to the pan. Toss to mix. Cook for a minute and check the seasoning. Add the basil and toss to mix again. Remove from the heat and set aside.

6. Remove the herbs and scallion greens from the quinoa. Fluff with a fork and tip onto a platter. Make a well in the center and tip the roasted ratatouille into it. Garnish with some basil leaves and serve.

## 5. Sweet Potato Muffins

Prep Time: 20 minutes

Cook Time: 35 minutes

Total Time: 55 minutes

Servings: 16

Ingredients

- 14 ounces (about 2 medium) sweet potato, washed with skins on
- 4 large eggs
- 2/3 cup brown sugar
- 2 teaspoons lemon zest
- 1 heaping teaspoon freshly grated ginger (optional)
- 2½ cups whole wheat pastry flour
- ½ teaspoon sea salt
- 2 teaspoons baking powder
- ½ teaspoon ground cinnamon
- ½ cup olive oil, plus more for muffin tins
- ¼ cup unsweetened applesauce
- ½ cup chopped walnuts
- ½ cup golden raisins

Instructions

1. Preheat the oven to 350 degrees. Line muffin tins with paper cups or lightly grease with olive oil.

2. Grate the sweet potato with a food processor or box grater. Transfer to a large bowl and mix with eggs, sugar, lemon zest, and ginger, until well blended.

3. Add in the whole-wheat pastry flour, salt, baking powder, olive oil, applesauce, walnuts, and raisins. Mix just until well blended. Do not over mix!

4. Spoon into muffin tins, filling the tins just under the brim. Bake for 20-25 minutes. Test for doneness with a toothpick—the toothpick should have some pieces of muffin on it, but not raw. Transfer to a wire rack and allow to cool slightly before eating.

## 6. Mushroom & Potato Breakfast Casserole

Prep Time: 1 hour

Cook Time: 55 minutes

Total Time: 1 hour 55 minutes

Servings: 6

Ingredients

- 2 Tablespoons olive oil
- ¼cup sliced bell pepper
- 1 cup quartered button mushrooms
- 3 baked Yukon gold or russet potatoes, diced (about three cups)
- ¼cup mixed chopped fresh herbs (parsley, dill, basil, etc.)
- 12 eggs
- Salt

Instructions

1. Preheat oven to 325 degrees F. Spray a 9x9 inch casserole dish with cooking spray or

2. In a large sauté pan, heat olive oil over a medium plan. Add the peppers and mushrooms. Season the

vegetables with a pinch of salt. Cook 2-3 minutes, until mushrooms are brown and peppers are tender.

3. Beat eggs.

4. Mix vegetables and potatoes into the casserole dish, sprinkle with herbs.

5. Pour eggs over the mixture and season with salt and pepper. Place the casserole dish on the center rack of the oven. Bake 20 minutes or until eggs are set in the center of the dish and the edges are golden brown.

## 7. Cheesy Swiss Chard & Egg Breakfast Tacos

Prep Time: 20 minutes

Cook Time: 35 minutes

Total Time: 55 minutes

Servings: 4

Ingredients

- 3 cups chopped Swiss chard, leaves only stems reserved for another use.
- ¼ cup sliced red onion
- 1 tablespoon extra virgin olive oil
- 4 eggs
- ½ cup shredded part-skim mozzarella cheese
- 12 small corn tortillas
- ¼ cup minced cilantro
- salt and pepper to taste

Instructions

1. In a non-stick sauté pan over medium heat, heat oil and add red onion. Cook until translucent. Add Swiss chard and cook for 3 to 5 minutes, or until slightly wilted. Add salt and pepper. Remove and reserve chard. Wipe pan.

2. In a small bowl, whisk eggs with salt and pepper.

3. Spray pan with cooking spray and place over medium low heat. Add eggs and cook until set and scrambled.

4. In a separate dry sauté pan over medium low heat, place one tortilla at a time in the pan to heat through.

5. Place a portion of Swiss chard, eggs, and cheese on each taco. Garnish with cilantro and serve.

## 8. Breakfast Strata (Savory Bread Pudding)

Prep Time: 45 minutes

Cook Time: 1 hour

Total Time: 1 hour 45 minutes

Servings: 6

Ingredients

- 1 tablespoon olive oil
- 12 ounces low sodium turkey sausage links
- 2 bell peppers, chopped (about 2 cups)
- 1 onion, chopped (about 2 cups)
- 1 12-ounce package frozen chopped spinach, thawed
- 12 eggs
- 4 cups skim milk
- 2 cups low fat shredded cheddar cheese
- 1 loaf sliced whole wheat bread, chopped
- salt and pepper to taste

Instructions

1. Preheat oven to 375 degrees. Spray a 9x13-inch casserole dish with cooking spray.

2. In a large sauté pan over medium heat, add olive oil. Add turkey sausage to pan, and brown on all sides. Once cooked, remove from pan and allow to cool. Chop sausage into bite sized pieces.

3. In same pan, add bell peppers and onion. Sauté for about 15 minutes, or until soft. Add spinach and cook for about 5 minutes. Season with salt and pepper. Add chopped sausage to pan and cool.

4. In a large bowl, combine eggs, milk and cheese. Season with a pinch of salt and pepper. Whisk egg mixture until combined. Add bread to egg mixture and allow bread to soak. Add cooled vegetables and stir to combine.

5. Pour bread and vegetable mixture into casserole pan, making sure to flatten the top into an even layer.

6. Place casserole in oven, and bake for about 45 minutes, until eggs are set and middle is firm.

## 9. Dutch Baby with Raspberry-Peach Compote

Prep Time: 20 minutes

Cook Time: 35 minutes

Total Time: 55 minutes

Servings: 4

Ingredients

- 3 peaches, pitted and sliced
- 2 cups raspberries
- ¼ cup sugar
- ⅓ cup coconut water (or water)
- ¼ cup raisins
- ¼ cup dried apricots, chopped
- 2 teaspoons lemon zest
- 3 eggs
- ⅔ cup whole milk
- ⅔ cup whole wheat flour
- ¼ teaspoon vanilla extract
- ¼ teaspoon cinnamon
- ⅛ teaspoon salt
- 1 stick butter, cut into pieces

Instructions

1. Preheat oven to 450F. Place cast iron skillet in oven to preheat.

2. To make compote, place a medium saucepan over high heat. Combine peaches, raspberries, sugar and coconut water in pan. Bring to boil, then lower to simmer. Cook for 10 minutes, until all fruit is soft.

3. Add raisins and dried apricots and cook for about 5 minutes, until fruit is rehydrated. Remove from heat and stir in lemon zest.

4. In a large bowl, whisk eggs thoroughly, about 2 minutes. Add milk, flour, vanilla, cinnamon and salt and whisk into the eggs. The batter should be thin.
5. Carefully remove the hot skillet from oven and add butter. Swirl skillet so the butter coats entire bottom. Quickly pour batter into skillet.

6. Bake for 18-20 minutes, or until golden brown and puffy.

7. Once baked, top with compote to serve.

## 10. Chicken Sausage & Vegetable Breakfast Casserole

Prep Time: 45 mniutes

Cook Time: 30 minutes

Total Time: 1 hour 15 minutes

Servings: 6

Ingredients

- 2 tablespoons olive oil
- 2 chicken sausages, sliced,
- 1 bell pepper, sliced
- ½ large yellow onion, sliced
- ¾ cup cherry tomatoes, halved
- 1 cup arugula
- ¼ cup chopped fresh herbs (e.g. parsley, chives, basil, etc.)
- 12 large eggs, whisked together

Instruction

1. Preheat oven to 325 degrees F. Prepare a 9x9 casserole dish by spraying it with cooking spray.

2. In a large skillet, heat olive oil over medium heat. Add the chicken sausage to the pan and cook until lightly

browned, about 5 minutes. Remove the sausage from pan with a slotted spoon and drain on paper towels.

3. Add the pepper and onion to the pan and season with a pinch of salt. Sauté the vegetables for about 5 to 10 minutes, or until the onions become translucent and turn slightly brown. Remove pan from heat.

4. Arrange the chicken sausage, peppers, onions, tomatoes, arugula, and herbs in the bottom of the casserole dish. Pour the whisked eggs on top of the vegetables.

5. Place the casserole dish in the center rack of the oven. Bake 20 minutes or until eggs are set in the center of the dish.

# LUNCH

## 11. Grilled Chicken Breasts in Rosemary Marinade

Prep Time: 20 minutes

Cook Time: 35 minutes

Total Time: 55 minutes

Servings: 4

Ingredients

Marinade:

- 2 tablespoons extra virgin olive oil
- 2 medium sprigs rosemary, leaves stripped and roughly chopped
- 2 cloves garlic, smashed and roughly chopped
- 1 teaspoon lemon zest
- Juice of 1 large lemon

Chicken:

- 2 skinless, whole chicken breasts, halved
- ⅓ cup water
- Salt, to taste

Instructions

1. Mix together all the marinade ingredients.

2. Place the chicken in a baking dish that"s large enough to hold all the pieces tightly. Pour the marinade over the chicken, turning it to make sure it is well coated. Cover and leave in the fridge for an hour, longer if you can, turning the pieces from time to time.

3. Heat the grill or broiler.

4. Turn the chicken in the marinade one more time to coat it evenly and set it on a plate. Sprinkle with a little sea salt.
5. Grill the chicken 5-8 minutes a side, depending on the thickness of the breasts. When it"s done, the juices should run clear. Let them sit a minute or two before serving.

6. Put the remaining marinade in a small saucepan. Add ⅓ cup water and a pinch of salt. Bring to a boil and cook down, stirring, until the mixture has reduced by about half.

7. Slice the breasts crossways and drizzle the sauce over them through a small strainer. Serve!

## 12. Roasted Fall Veggie Vegan Tacos

Prep Time: 15 minutes

Cook Time: 30 minutes

Total Time: 45 minutes

Servings: 4

Ingredients

- 1 small butternut squash, diced into ½" cubes (about 4 cups)
- 1 small cauliflower, cut into medium florets
- 2 tablespoons extra-virgin olive oil
- 12 small corn tortillas
- 1 ripe avocado, cut into 12 slices
- 2 tablespoons minced cilantro
- salt and pepper to taste
- lime wedges

Instructions:

1. Preheat oven to 375 degrees.

2. On a baking sheet lined with parchment paper place butternut squash and cauliflower. Drizzle with olive

oil and sprinkle with salt and pepper. Bake for 30 minutes or until vegetables are golden brown.

3. Meanwhile, in a dry sauté pan over medium low heat, place one tortilla at a time in the pan to heat through. Keep warm in foil at the back of the stove.

4. Assemble tacos by placing a piece of avocado on each warm tortilla and smashing it onto bottom of the tortilla with a fork. Season with salt and pepper. Top the avocado with roasted vegetables and cilantro. Serve immediately with lime wedges.

## 13. Lemon-Soy Baked Tofu Steaks

Prep Time: 20 minutes

Cook Time: 35 minutes

Total Time: 55 minutes

Servings: 8

Ingredients

- 2 blocks of firm tofu, sliced into ½-inch thick slices.

Marinade:

- ⅔ cup soy sauce
- 2 teaspoon grated lemon zest
- 4 tablespoons lemon juice
- 2 tablespoons balsamic vinegar
- 2 teaspoons sugar
- 4 tablespoons olive oil
- 2 cloves garlic, crushed and sliced
- 2 tablespoon chopped fresh herbs – I suggest tarragon, rosemary or thyme (Optional)

Instructions

1. Lay the tofu out on a board or tray lined with paper towels or a clean tea towel. Cover with more paper. Lay a wooden cutting board or other weight on top to press out the excess moisture so that the marinade won't be diluted. (I often use wine or water bottles as weights.) This will take about 30 minutes. It's best to do this near the sink. You will be amazed by how much water comes out.

2. Preheat the oven to 400 degrees.

3. Put all the ingredients together in a saucepan, except the herbs. Bring to a boil. Take it off the heat immediately and cool. Add the herbs once the marinade is off the heat.

4. Once the tofu is drained, pat the slices dry. Spoon a little marinade onto a lightly greased baking dish and lay the tofu slices over it, side by side in a single layer. Pour the rest of the marinade over them. Bake uncovered for 25 minutes, turning the slices over about halfway through. The tofu should be brown and

almost dry, and any remaining marinade thick and syrupy. Serve immediately!

## 14. Thai-Style Tempeh Curry

Prep Time: 30 minutes

Cook Time: 25 minutes

Total Time: 55 minutes

Servings: 4

Ingredients

- 1 (8-ounce) block tempeh
- 2 tablespoons canola or grapeseed oil
- 1 teaspoon whole coriander seeds
- 1 clove of garlic, thinly sliced
- 1 jalapeño pepper, seeded and sliced into thin strips (optional)
- 1-inch piece of ginger, peeled and cut into julienne
- 1 large onion, halved and thinly sliced through the root end
- 2 carrots, julienned
- 1 medium Italian frying or bell pepper, seeded and cut into julienne strips
- ½ a small Savoy cabbage (about 1lb), cored, the thickest stems cut away, then finely shredded
- ½ teaspoon turmeric

- ½ teaspoon ground coriander
- ¼ teaspoon cayenne, or to taste
- 1 (14-ounce) can light coconut milk
- ½ cup water
- 1 tablespoon Thai fish sauce or sea salt, to taste
- 1 to 2 teaspoons toasted sesame oil
- Juice of 1 lime
- 3 tablespoons roughly chopped cilantro leaves

Instructions

1. Broil or grill the tempeh until it is well browned all over. When it is cool enough to handle, cut diagonally into slices about ¼-inch thick. Set aside.

2. Heat the oil in a wok or wide sauté pan over medium-high heat. When the oil starts to shimmer, add the coriander seeds and fry for a few seconds until they start to darken. Then add the garlic, jalapeño, and ginger. Stir-fry until the garlic starts to color slightly. Add the onions, carrots, and Italian pepper, and stir-fry until they begin to soften but not brown.

3. Add half the shredded cabbage. Stir-fry the cabbage until it starts to soften, then add the tempeh slices and

gently mix in with the veggies. Cook for a minute. Add the turmeric, ground coriander, and cayenne, and mix to coat the tempeh and vegetables. Cook, stirring, for a minute. Do not let the spices burn.

4. Add the remaining cabbage, coconut milk, ¼ cup of water (use it to rinse out the coconut milk stuck in the can), salt or fish sauce, and sesame oil. Mix well. Cover and turn the heat down to simmer.

5. Cook for about 10-15 minutes or until cabbage is tender, checking that nothing is sticking. Add some more water if looks too dry. It should be saucy but not swimming. When the cabbage is cooked, remove cover, add the lime juice and cilantro, and mix well. Adjust seasonings. Cook for another minute. It's ready!

## 15. Persian New Year Noodle Soup

Prep Time: 30 minutes

Cook Time: 25 minutes

Total Time: 55 minutes

Servings: 6

Ingredients

- 7 tablespoons olive oil
- 2 bunches scallions, chopped
- 3 cloves garlic, minced
- 1 teaspoon ground turmeric
- 10 cups low-sodium vegetable or chicken stock
- ¼ cup dried lentils, picked through and washed.
- ½ cup fresh flat-leaf parsley, chopped
- ½ cup fresh cilantro, chopped
- 2 cups packed leafy greens (spinach, kale), thick stems removed and coarsely chopped
- Salt, to taste
- 6 ounces whole wheat spaghettini, broken into quarters
- 2 yellow onions, cut in half and thinly sliced
- 1 large handful fresh mint leaves, finely chopped

- ½ cup canned chickpeas, drained and rinsed
- ¼ cup canned kidney beans, drained and rinsed
- ½ cup canned navy beans, drained and rinsed
- 2 cups plain Greek yogurt, for garnish (optional)

Instructions

1. Heat a large pot over medium-high heat 4 tablespoons of the olive oil with scallions and garlic. Cook for 3 minutes or until the garlic starts to soften.

2. Add the turmeric. Cook for a minute to blend the flavors. Add the lentils, parsley, cilantro, spinach, and a pinch of salt. Stir to mix. Add the stock, bring to a boil then turn the heat down to a simmer. Cook for 20 minutes. Add the spaghettini. Simmer for 10 minutes more.

3. Meanwhile, over a medium high flame, heat the remaining 3 tablespoons of olive oil in a frying pan and fry the onions until golden brown, about 8-10 minutes. Add the mint and cook 1 minute more. Set aside.

4. Add chickpeas, kidney beans, and navy beans to the soup and continue to simmer for 10 minutes. Taste for salt. The soup is ready. Serve with a dollop of yogurt and fried onions.

## 16. Warm Quinoa Salad with Sofrito

Prep Time: 30 minutes

Cook Time: 50 minutes

Total Time: 1 hour 20 minutes

Servings: 6

Ingredients

- 2 cups quinoa, rinsed well in a fine sieve
- 3 tablespoons chopped Italian parsley, plus 1 sprig
- 1½ tablespoons finely chopped cilantro, plus 1 sprig
- 1 teaspoon plus 2 tablespoons olive oil
- 4 cups water or stock
- 3 medium shallots, finely chopped
- 2 tablespoons torn basil or mint leaves (optional)
- 2 small orange peppers, deseeded and cut into a small dice
- 4 small zucchini, cut into a small dice
- Sea salt, to taste
- 1 teaspoon ground cumin
- Grated zest of 1 small lemon
- 4 scallions white parts finely chopped, green tops reserved

Instructions

1. Put the quinoa, parsley sprig, cilantro sprig, and scallion greens into a saucepan with a lid. Add the 4 cups of water and t teaspoon of olive oil. Bring to a boil, then cover, turn heat down to low and simmer for 20 minutes. Take off the heat and set aside, covered until you are ready to use it.

2. Meanwhile, make the sofrito. Heat the remaining 2 tablespoons of olive oil in a large sauté pan over medium heat. Add the shallots and gently sauté for 2-3 minutes or until they start to soften. Add the peppers and zucchini, cook for another 2-3 minutes until they start to soften. Add salt to taste, turn the heat down and partially cover. Continue to cook until the shallots have started to caramelize and the other vegetables are very soft, about 10-15 minutes.

3. Remove the herbs and scallion greens from the quinoa. Fluff with a fork.

4. Remove the cover from the vegetables. Turn up to medium-high and add the ground cumin. Cook, stirring for 1 minute, then add the chopped parsley,

cilantro, scallions, and lemon zest. Stir to mix well and cook for a minute to blend the flavors. Add the quinoa, a little at a time until the dish is about ½ quinoa ½ vegetables. Stir to mix. Just before serving, add the torn basil or mint leaves. Serve immediately.

## 17. Fish 'en Papillote' with Ginger & Coconut

Prep Time: 20 minutes

Cook Time: 45 minutes

Total Time: 55 minutes

Servings: 4

Ingredients

- ¼ cup fresh squeezed lime juice
- 2 small garlic cloves, thinly sliced lengthways
- ½-inch piece fresh ginger root, peeled and grated
- 2 shallots, thinly sliced
- 1 small red pepper, deseeded, deveined and thinly sliced into julienne sticks
- ¼ pound green beans, halved and quartered into julienne strips
- 2 (6-ounce) fillets of red snapper or cod
- ¼ teaspoon turmeric powder
- ½ teaspoon ground coriander
- 2 teaspoons olive oil, divided
- 2 sprigs cilantro plus 2 tablespoons chopped for garnish
- Salt, to taste

- 3 tablespoons coconut milk

Instructions

1. Mix the lime juice, garlic and ginger together. Coat the fish fillets with it and let it sit and marinate for 30 minutes.

2. Meanwhile, preheat the oven to 400 degrees.

3. Tear off 2 squares of aluminum foil large enough to comfortably hold 1 fish fillet. If lining your packets with parchment paper, cut pieces the same size as the foil, and lay it on top of the matte side of the foil.

4. Toss the shallots, red pepper, and green beans together. Divide into two equal portions.
5. Remove the fish from the marinade, reserving the remaining marinade. Diagonally slash the skin of each fish fillet 3 times. Rub the fillets with the turmeric and coriander.

6. Smear the center of each foil/parchment square with 1 teaspoon oil. Then lay equal amounts of shallots, red pepper, and green beans, onto the foil. Spoon half of

the remaining marinade over each vegetable pile. Top the vegetables with a fish fillet, skin side up, then lay the sprig of cilantro over it and sprinkle with a pinch of salt.

7. Fold the foil in half over the fish and tightly roll the sides of the packet together to seal, leaving a small gap open. Mix the coconut milk and remaining marinade. Pour equal amounts of this mixture through the gap into each packet and then finish sealing them. The packet should have the look of a giant empanada or calzone.

8. Lay the packets on a cookie sheet and bake in the oven 10-15 minutes depending on the thickness of the fish.

9. Carefully open the packets, there will be steam. Discard the sprig of cilantro. Sprinkle with chopped cilantro and serve in the half open packets, or plate the vegetables with the fish.

## 18. Mushroom Burger

Prep Time: 15 minutes

Cook Time: 35 minutes

Total Time: 50 minutes

Servings: 4

Ingredients

- 4 (4 to 5-inch diameter) portabella mushroom caps, wiped
- 1 cup grape or cherry tomatoes, sliced in half lengthwise
- 2 tablespoons olive oil
- Salt and pepper, to taste
- 6-ounces mozzarella, cut into 4 slices
- 4 whole wheat burger buns
- Handful of arugula

For the Basil Pesto:

- 1 clove of garlic
- 1/2 cup of pine nuts, toasted until golden and cooled
- 1/2 cup grated Parmesan cheese
  - cups sweet basil leaves, washed

- Sea salt and pepper, to taste
- 1/4 cup extra virgin olive oil

Instructions

1. Preheat the broiler. Make the basil pesto as outlined here.

2. Spread the mushroom caps, rounded side down, and the tomatoes, cut side up on a baking tray. Drizzle with olive oil, salt and pepper.

3. Place 6-inches under the broiler for 7 minutes. Lay the cheese on the mushroom caps, and continue to broil until melted, about 2 minutes. Remove from oven, then lightly toast the burger buns under the broiler.
4. Lay the buns open on a work surface and spread a heaping tablespoon of Basil Pesto on the bottom bun. Evenly divide the tomatoes between the four buns and place the mushrooms on them cheesy side down. Top with arugula and the top bun and serve.

## 19. Asparagus & Goat Cheese Frittata

Prep Time: 30 minutes

Cook Time: 35 minutes

Total Time: 1 hour 5 minutes

Servings: 4

Ingredients

- 4 large eggs
- ¼ cup water
- 1 tablespoon freshly grated Parmesan cheese
- Salt and pepper, to taste
- 2 teaspoons extra virgin olive oil
- 1 tablespoon chopped scallions, white and light green parts only
- ½-pound steamed asparagus, cut into ½-inch pieces, tips reserved.
- 1 medium potato boiled, cut into a ½-inch dice
- 2-ounce fresh goat cheese log crumbled
- Olive oil or unsalted butter, as needed

Instructions

1. Preheat the oven to 350 degrees.

2. In a large bowl, whisk the eggs. Gradually beat in the water. Add the Parmesan, salt and pepper to taste.

3. Heat the olive oil in a skillet over medium heat, Sauté the scallions until soft. Put the scallion mixture into the egg mixture.

4. Grease the skillet with a little butter or olive oil. Arrange the reserved asparagus tips in the bottom of the pan. Set aside.

5. Mix the remaining cut asparagus and potato pieces into the eggs and herbs. Fold in the goat cheese. Carefully pour the egg mixture over the asparagus tips in the skillet. Put the skillet in the middle of the oven and bake until the frittata is set, about 35 to 40 minutes. Let cool for 5 minutes in the pan. Turn the frittata out onto a plate to cool to room temperature. Serve with a simple green salad.

## 20. Lemon-Soy Marinated Chicken

Prep Time: 20 minutes

Cook Time: 35 minutes

Total Time: 55 minutes

Servings: 8

Ingredients

- 1 whole chicken, skin on, cut into 8 pieces

Marinade:

- ⅔ cup soy sauce
- 2 tablespoons balsamic vinegar
- 2 teaspoons sugar
- 2 tablespoons olive oil
- 2 cloves garlic, crushed and sliced
- 4 tablespoons lemon juice
- 2 teaspoon grated lemon zest
- 2 tablespoons chopped fresh herbs, I would use tarragon, rosemary or thyme (optional)

Instructions

1. Put all the marinade ingredients except the herbs together in a saucepan. Bring the mixture to a boil. Take it off the heat immediately, add the herbs and let it cool.

2. Pat the chicken pieces dry and lay them in a dish in one layer. Cover with the marinade. Leave the chicken to sit in the marinade for at least 1 hour in the refrigerator, turning the pieces every so often to make sure they are marinating evenly.

3. Preheat the oven to 400 degrees. Transfer marinated chicken to an oven-safe baking sheet, cover with aluminum foil, and bake for 20 to 25 minutes, basting with remaining marinade every 8-10 minutes, until internal temperature reaches 165 degrees fahrenheit. Remove chicken from the oven.
4. Turn oven broiler on. When broiler is ready, put chicken in oven and broil until skin is lightly browned, about 3-5 minutes. Remove from oven and let rest for 5 to 10 minutes before serving.

# DINNERS

## 21. Chicken Taco Dinner

Prep Time: 30 minutes

Cook Time: 45 minutes

Total Time: 1 hour 15 minutes

Servings: 6

Ingredients

- 1½ pounds chicken breast
- ½ medium onion
- 1 clove garlic, smashed
- Salt, to taste, divided
- 1 small head of romaine lettuce, washed, shredded and patted dry
- ¾ cup thinly sliced radishes
- 2 teaspoons olive oil
- 1 teaspoon white wine vinegar
- 1 avocado, halved and pitted
- 3 limes, divided
- ½ red onion, thinly sliced
- 12 6 inch corn tortillas
- 1 cup fresh cilantro, washed

- ¾ cup queso fresco
- Salsa Verde or tomato salsa (optional)

Instructions

1. In a stockpot, cover the chicken, onion, and garlic with water by 1-inch. Add 1 teaspoon of salt and bring to a boil. Reduce heat and simmer for 30-40 minutes. Once cool enough to handle, shred the chicken with fingers and season to taste.

2. Meanwhile, prep all the vegetables. Toss the romaine and the radishes with oil, vinegar, salt and pepper. Pour into a bowl. Smash the avocado with juice from 1 lime, some salt and pepper, and transfer to a serving bowl. Set the sliced red onions onto a small plate. Cut the remaining limes into wedges.
3. Warm the tortillas one at a time in an ungreased skillet or wrapped in foil in the oven. Cover with a paper towel and set on the table along with the shredded chicken, salad, cilantro, avocado, limes, queso fresco, and corn tortillas. Allow everyone to assemble their tacos as desired.

## 22. Cauliflower Spoonbread

Prep Time: 20 minutes

Cook Time: 50 minutes

Total Time: 1 hour 10 minutes

Servings: 4

Ingredients

- 1 medium cauliflower, rinsed and trimmed
- 1½ cups whole or 2% milk
- 2 to 3 cardamom pods or to taste
- 1 bay leaf
- Salt
- 1 tablespoon unsalted butter
- 2 eggs separated, plus 1 egg white
- ½ cup crumbled feta cheese
- Pinch of cream of tartar

Instructions

1. Preheat oven to 375°F. Grease a 2-quart, deep-sided baking dish or soufflé dish.

2. Break the cauliflower into florets. Set ½ cup of florets aside to be used in Step 3. Combine the milk, cardamom pods, bay leaf, and ½ teaspoon salt in a pot and bring to a boil. Add the florets, partially cover, and reduce the heat to a simmer. Cook until florets are soft, about 10 minutes. Remove pot from the heat.

3. Reserve ½ cup of the milk and discard the cardamom and bay leaf. Put the cauliflower into a blender with 1/2 cup of the cooking milk and blend until puréed. (Use caution when blending hot liquids.) Taste for salt. Let cool slightly. Add the egg yolks and blend at high speed and pour into a large bowl.

4. While the florets are simmering, heat the butter in a small frying pan. Take the reserved cauliflower and roughly chop. Fry in the butter until soft and golden. Fold into the cauliflower purée along with two-thirds of the feta cheese.
5. In a medium bowl, beat the egg whites and cream of tartar until stiff peaks form. Take a spoonful and add it to the cauliflower to break up the purée. Add in the rest and gently fold into the cauliflower mixture. Scrape into the prepared dish, sprinkle with the

remaining feta and bake for 40 minutes, or until puffy and golden. Eat immediately

## 23. Mushroom Empanadas

Prep Time: 45 minutes

Cook Time: 50 minutes

Total Time: 1 hour 35 minutes

Servings: 4

Ingredients

For Dough

- 2 cups all-purpose flour
- 1 teaspoon salt
- 1/2 cup olive oil
- 1 tablespoon white vinegar
- 2 eggs

For Filling

- 2 cups cooked sliced mushrooms
- 1 cup sautéed chopped onions
- ½ cup shredded mozzarella cheese

Instructions

1. Preheat oven to 350 degrees. Line baking sheet with parchment paper.

2. In a large bowl, add flour and salt, stir to combine. Make a well in the center and add olive oil, distilled vinegar and eggs.

3. Using a wooden spoon, stir wet ingredients into dry ingredients until a dough forms. Turn out onto a work surface and knead until smooth. If dough is too dry, add 1 tablespoon of water. Cover with plastic wrap and rest for 1 hour.

4. Meanwhile, to make chimichurri, combine red wine vinegar, garlic, cumin red pepper flakes and parsley in the bowl of a food processor and blend until a paste forms. With the motor running, slowly drizzle in olive oil until incorporated. Season with salt and pepper. Pour into a small bowl and reserve.
5. On a floured worked surface, roll dough out until it is a ¼ inch thick. Using a 4-inch round cookie cutter, cut out circles of the dough. (The scraps can be rolled out one more time to prevent waste).

6. Fill each dough round with about a tablespoon of mushrooms, portion of onions and cheese.

7. Using a pastry brush, brush water around the edge of the dough. Fold the edges together to create a half moon. Crimp edges with a fork to seal and poke a hole in the top with a fork so steam can escape.

8. Place on baking sheet and spray empanadas with cooking spray.

9. Bake for 20-25 minutes or until dough is lightly golden brown.

10. Serve with chimichurri.

## 23. Fusili with Roast Vegetables & Romesco

Prep Time: 30 minutes

Cook Time: 55 minutes

Total Time: 1 hour 25 minutes

Servings: 6

Ingredients

- 3 cups diced eggplant, about 1 medium
- 3 medium red peppers, deseeded
- ½ cup halved cherry tomatoes
- 1 medium shallot, sliced
- 4 cloves garlic, kept in its peel
- 1 tablespoon olive oil
- Salt and pepper, to taste
- 6 ounces whole-wheat fusilli
- 6 cups baby spinach leaves
- 3 tablespoons almonds
- 2 tablespoons red wine vinegar
- 3 tablespoons Parmesan cheese
- ¼ cup olive oil
- 6 small fresh mozzarella balls halved, or half of 1 large ball, cut into a ½-inch dice

Instructions

1. Preheat the oven to 425 degrees.

2. In a large bowl, toss the eggplant, red peppers, cherry tomatoes, shallot and garlic with 1 tablespoon of olive oil, salt and pepper, to taste. Spread onto a baking sheet in a single layer. Roast for 20 minutes or until tender and well browned. When the vegetables are done, allow them to cool slightly. Set half of the peppers to one side for the dressing.

3. Meanwhile, bring a large stockpot full of water to a boil. Add the fusili and a large pinch of salt. Cook for 3 minutes less than the package instructions, add in the spinach and cook for 1 more minute. Drain well, drizzle with olive oil, and let cool at room temperature, turning every so often.

4. To make the Romesco dressing, take the cooled roasted red peppers you set aside, and puree with the almonds, red wine vinegar, Parmesan cheese, and olive oil. Taste for seasonings.

5. Toss the cooled pasta, spinach and the roasted vegetables with the dressing. Stir in the fresh mozzarella. Eat at room temperature or cover and keep in the refrigerator until ready to eat.

## 24. Chicken Sausage & Chestnut Stuffing

Prep Time: 30 minutes

Cook Time: 55 minutes

Total Time: 1 hour 25 minutes

Servings: 4

Ingredients

- 2 tablespoons olive oil
- 12 ounces hot Italian or breakfast-style chicken sausage, about 4 links, casings removed
- 4 cups whole wheat French-style bread, cut into ¼-inch cubes, lightly toasted
- ¼ cup (4 tablespoons) butter, divided
- 1 cup chopped onion
- 1 cup diced celery
- 2 tablespoons fresh sage leaves, sliced
- 1 tablespoon fresh thyme leaves
- ¼ cup chopped fresh parsley
- Salt, to taste
- 3 cups chopped kale
- 1 cup halved chestnuts
- ½ cup broth, plus more if needed

- 2 large eggs, lightly whisked

Instructions

1. Preheat the oven to 375 degrees.

2. Heat the olive oil in a large wide skillet over medium-high heat. Add the sausage, breaking up with a wooden spoon, until golden and cooked through, about 5 minutes. Using a slotted spoon remove the sausage and put into a large bowl with the toasted bread cubes. Set aside.

3. In the same skillet melt 2 tablespoons of the butter over medium heat, scraping up any of the sausage remains. Add the onion, celery, sage, thyme, parsley and a generous pinch of salt. Cook for 8 to 10 minutes, or until the onion is translucent and just beginning to brown.

4. Add the chopped kale, and cook, stirring until well wilted, about 3 minutes. Pour this mixture into the bowl with the sausage and bread.

5. Stir in the chestnuts, taste for seasoning, then mix in the broth and whisked eggs until well combined.

6. Transfer the stuffing mixture to a baking dish, dot with the remaining 2 tablespoons of butter and cover with foil. Bake for 30 minutes, then remove foil and bake for another 20 minutes, adding more broth or water if it looks too dry. Serve with our Basic Roast Turkey or Chicken.

## 25. Cider Glazed Turkey

Prep Time: 30 minutes

Cook Time: 55 minutes

Total Time: 1 hour 25 minutes

Servings: 12

Ingredients

For the turkey:

- 1 (12 pound) turkey
- ¼ cup olive oil
- Salt and pepper, to taste
- 2 apples, cut into chunks
- 5 sprigs of rosemary
- 1 onion, quartered

For the glaze:

- 1½ cups apple cider
- 1 tablespoon sugar (optional)
- 2 sprigs rosemary
- ½ cup butter

For the gravy:

- 2 tablespoons butter
- ¼ cup flour
- 2 cups stock
- 2 cups water or Martinelli's non-alcoholic cider

Instructions

1. Preheat the oven to 425 degrees.

2. Remove the giblets from the turkey. Transfer to a roasting pan. Rub the olive oil all over the turkey, and rub in a generous amount of salt and pepper all over.
3. Put the apple, rosemary and onion into the cavity of the turkey. Tie the drumsticks together with kitchen twine and tuck the wings underneath the body.

4. Roast in the oven for 30 minutes. Pour in 1 cup of water or stock into the pan and cover the turkey very loosely with foil. Reduce the heat to 325 degrees. Cook for another hour.

5. While the turkey is roasting, in a small saucepan combine the apple cider, sugar and rosemary sprig. Cook over low heat, until reduced to about ¼ cup, about 8 to 10 minutes. Discard the rosemary and

remove from heat. Whisk in the butter 1 tablespoon at a time. Set aside, keeping warm, until ready to use.

6. When the inside of the turkey reads between 165 and 170 degrees, remove from the oven and let sit for 15 minutes before carving. Serve with the gravy.

## 26. Fall Vegetable Soup with Spicy Gremolata

Prep Time: 20 minutes

Cook Time: 30 minutes

Total Time: 50 minutes

Servings: 8

Ingredients

- 1 whole dried chipotle pepper pod, or ½ teaspoon of dried chipotle
- 1-pound kabocha or butter cup squash, seeded, and diced
- ½-pound onions or leeks, finely sliced
- 2 carrots, scrubbed and diced
- 6 garlic cloves, crushed and peeled
- 1-pound Yukon Gold potatoes, scrubbed, quartered lengthwise, and sliced to form a dice
- ½-pound green beans, topped, tailed, cut into ¾-inch lengths
- ½-pound zucchini, quartered lengthwise and thickly sliced to form a dice (optional)
- 1 bouquet garni
- 2 teaspoons sea salt

- 2 (14-ounce) cans of cannellini beans, drained and rinsed
- 1 cup small whole wheat elbow macaroni
- Freshly grated Parmesan, to taste (optional)
- Pepper, to taste
- 1 recipe Spicy Gremolata

Instructions

1. Place all of the soup vegetables into a large pot, except for the canned beans and the macaroni.

2. Add the bouquet garni and 3 quarts of water, or enough to cover the vegetables by 1-inch. Add the salt. Bring to a boil, cover and let simmer gently for an hour or until the vegetables are tender and the squash can be mashed against the sides of the pan. While the soup is cooking, prepare the Spicy Gremolata (to learn how, click here).
3. Remove the bouquet garni. Mash some of the squash against the pan to thicken the broth. Add the beans, cook for 10 minutes. Taste for salt. Add the macaroni. Cook until al dente. Stir in the Spicy Herb Pesto and serve immediately with the grated cheese.

## 27. Winter Squash Risotto

Prep Time: 20 minutes

Cook Time: 45 minutes

Total Time: 1 hour 5 minutes

Servings: 4

Ingredients

- 1 tablespoon olive oil
- 1 small yellow onion, chopped
- 3 pounds kabocha or butternut squash seeded, peeled and cut into a 1-inch dice
- 4 cups plus 2 cups hot water or low sodium vegetable stock
- 2 cups Arborio rice
- 2 tablespoons freshly grated Parmesan cheese, or to taste
- 2 tablespoons butter, or to taste
- 1 clove garlic, thinly sliced
- 8 to 10 large, fresh sage leaves, shredded
- Sea salt, to taste

Instructions

1. Heat the olive oil in a Dutch oven over medium heat. Add the onion, sprinkle with salt and cook until it starts to soften, about 4 to 5 minutes. Add the pumpkin, stir to mix. Cover and sweat over a medium heat for 8 minutes, stirring from time to time, or until the pumpkin has started to soften.

2. Add 4 cups of stock, bring to a boil and cover. Lower the heat and simmer for 15 minutes, or until the pumpkin is soft. Add the rice, stir to mix and cook for 15 minutes. The pumpkin will have disintegrated and the rice just al dente. Add a little extra stock if it looks very thick. Stir in the Parmesan. Taste for salt.

3. While the rice is cooking, melt the butter in a small pan or skillet over a low flame. Do this slowly for the best results. When the butter has stopped foaming and is clear with nut-brown residue, add the garlic and cook until it is just golden. Remove, and turn up the heat a notch and add the shredded sage leaves. Cook until just crisp, about 2 minutes. Reserve half the leaves.

4. Stir the butter mixture into the rice. Cover and let sit for 2 minutes. Add a little extra warm stock if the risotto looks dry – it should be a little soupy. Serve immediately sprinkled with the reserved sage leaves and a chunk of Parmesan to grate over the top.

## 28. Roast Chicken with Olives, Shallots & Prunes

Prep Time: 30 minutes

Cook Time: 45 minutes

Total Time: 1 hour 15 minutes

Servings: 8

Ingredients

- 1 cup whole pitted green olives
- ½ cup prunes, quartered
- 4 medium shallots, quartered
- 1 large lemon, cut in half, then quartered
- 1 teaspoon olive oil
- Salt, to taste
- 2 teaspoons ground cumin
- 2 teaspoons salt
- 2 teaspoons paprika
- 1 teaspoon cayenne pepper
- ½ teaspoon turmeric
- 1 tablespoon olive oil
- 3 pound whole chicken, quartered
- 1 cup water
- 1 tablespoon red wine vinegar

- 1 bay leaf

Instructions

1. Preheat the oven to 350 degrees.

2. Spread the olives, prunes, shallots and lemon sliced in the bottom of a deep roasting pan. Drizzle with 1 teaspoon of olive oil and salt.

3. Mix the cumin, salt, paprika, cayenne and turmeric together. Rub evenly onto the chicken.
4. Heat 1 tablespoon of olive oil over medium-high in a wide skillet, brown the chicken in batches, turning to brown all sides. Place the chicken on top of the olive mixture in the roasting pan. Once all the chicken has been browned, add the 1 cup of water and 1 tablespoon of vinegar to the pan, over high heat scrape up the bits at the bottom of the pan and cook until half has evaporated. Pour this into the roasting pan.

5. Roast for 20 to 30 minutes or until all the chicken is cooked through. Let rest then serve with Basic Couscous.

## 29. Salmon Cakes with Dijon Yogurt Sauce

Prep Time: 30 minutes

Cook Time: 45 minutes

Total Time: 1 hour 15 minutes

Servings: 4

Ingredients

For salmon cakes:

- 2 tablespoons Greek yogurt
- 1 tablespoon lemon juice
- 1 ½ teaspoons Dijon mustard
- ¼ cup finely chopped green onion
- 2 tablespoons minced red bell pepper
- ½ teaspoon garlic powder
- ¼ teaspoon salt
- pinch cayenne
- 10 ounces of canned salmon, flaked, skin and bones removed
- 1 large egg, lightly beaten
- 1 cup panko
- 1 tablespoon canola oil

For sauce:

- 2 tablespoons Greek yogurt
- 1 teaspoon Dijon mustard
- 1 teaspoon lemon juice
- 1 tablespoon parsley, chopped
- 1 teaspoon capers, chopped
- ½ teaspoon garlic
- dash salt

Instructions

1. Mix together the yogurt, lemon juice and mustard. Add the green onion, red pepper, garlic powder, salt, cayenne, and salmon. Mix thoroughly.

2. Add the egg, mix thoroughly. Mix in the panko and form four equal size patties.

3. Heat the oil in a large non-stick skillet over medium-high heat, and cook the patties until brown, about 5 minutes on each side.

4. To make the sauce, mix together yogurt, mustard, lemon juice, parsley, capers, garlic and salt.
5. Spoon the sauce over the finished salmon cakes.

## 30. Italian Wedding Soup

Prep Time: 30 minutes

Cook Time: 45 minutes

Total Time: 1 hour 15 minutes

Servings: 6

Ingredients

- ¾-pound ground chicken
- ⅔ cup breadcrumbs
- 1 large egg
- ½ cup freshly grated Parmesan cheese
- 1 tablespoon fresh oregano, chopped
- 1 teaspoon lemon zest
- 1 garlic clove, minced
- ¼ teaspoon red pepper flakes (optional)
- Salt and pepper, to taste
- 1 tablespoon olive oil
- 4 cups chicken stock
- 6 kale leaves, stems removed, roughly chopped
- ¼ cup freshly grated Parmesan

Instructions

1. In a bowl, mix together the ground chicken, breadcrumbs, egg, Parmesan, oregano, lemon zest, garlic, red pepper flakes, salt and pepper. Form into 1-inch balls.

2. Heat 1 tablespoon of olive oil in a wide skillet over medium-high heat. Cook the meatballs until evenly golden brown, they do not need to be cooked all the way through as they will finish cooking in the soup. Transfer the meatballs to a plate covered with a plate lined with paper towels.

3. Heat the chicken stock and bring to a boil. Add the kale leaves and the meatballs. Simmer for 15 minutes. Stir in ¼ cup of Parmesan cheese. Taste the broth for seasonings then serve.

www.ingramcontent.com/pod-product-compliance
Ingram Content Group UK Ltd.
Pitfield, Milton Keynes, MK11 3LW, UK
UKHW022012190726
13853UKWH00004B/1887

9 798549 584815